Freedom In Locs

Amy McKnight

Copyright © 2022 by Amy McKnight Unlimitted LLC

All rights reserved.

No portion of this book may be reproduced in any form without written permission from the publisher or author, except as permitted by U.S. copyright law.

Contents

Who Should Read This Book	1
My Promise to You	5
Introduction	7
1. Getting Started With Your Why	11
Questions to Consider Before Starting	
Dealing with Family & Friends	
Reflections to Action	
2. The Best Installation Method for YOU!	15
What Are Locs?	
Hair Texture & Installation Methods	
Choosing an Installation Method	
Starting Locs with Coils	

Starting Locs with Two-Strand Twists
Starting Locs with Three-Strand Braids
Starting Locs By Interlocking
Starting Instant Locs
Loc Method + Hair Texture Chart
Reflection to Action

3. Instant Length with Permanent Loc Extensions   35
Before Getting Loc Extensions...
Methods of Extending Locs
Premade Permanent Lock Extensions
Installing Permanent Loc Extensions
Reflection to Action

4. Preparing Your Hair To Lock   49
Make Sure Your Hair is Long Enough
Getting a Clean Start
Loc Friendly Shampoos
Reflection to Action

5. Getting Your Sections Sorted   53
Parting Size Versus Eventual Loc Size
Micro-sized Isn't Necessarily the Best

    Loc Parting Styles
    Professional Parting Help is Worth It
    Consider Getting a Friend to Help You
    How to See the Back Of Your Head
    Reflection to Action

6. The Professional Loc Installation   65
    The Consultation
    The Lead-Up
    What to Bring & What Not to Bring
    After Locking Care
    Reflection to Action

7. Maintenance: Taking care of your investment   71
    Products, Products, Products
    Best Practices for Washing
    Suggestions for Separating
    Best Practices for Drying
    Afro-Kinky Hair Root Maintenance Methods
    Straight, Wavy, or Mixed Textured Hair
    Coloring Your Locs
    Covering Your Locs
    Swimming with Locs

Reflection to Action

8. Recipes for Healthy Dreads 87
    Conditioning with Natural Oils
    Herbs and Essential Oils
    Natural Hair Lightening & Coloring
    Acid Rinses
    Herbal Rinses & Refreshing Sprays

9. When Things Go Wrong 94
    Dissatisfaction with Your Locs
    Thinning/Weak Locs
    Mold in Your Locs
    Super Skinny Locs
    Loopy Bumpy Locs
    Frizzy Locks
    Uneven Locs
    Removing Locs

10. How We Help People Get Beautiful Locs 101
     We Give Educated Guidance
     We Share Informed Suggestions
     We Provide Empathetic Support

11. The Next Step — 104
    Don't Lose Your Momentum
    How to Schedule Our Call

Bibliography — 109

Acknowledgments — 112

Fullpage Image — 116

About Amy McKnight — 117

Also By Amy McKnight — 119

About the Freedom In Locs Podcast — 120

A Small Request — 121

Who Should Read This Book

This is an intentionally short book with all the fluff and filler removed, designed to be read in a single setting so you can gain insights as quickly as possible. Still, I don't want to waste your time if it is not a good fit. So, please take a few moments to read this entire section to see if the *Freedom in Locs* book is an intelligent investment of your time, energy, and focus. I wrote this short book for the following reasons:

> 1. To provide a concise and comprehensive guide on what it takes to start and maintain locs on

wavy, curly, coily, kinky, wiry, or mixed textured hair.

2. To provide a framework of best practices to avoid pitfalls if you plan to DIY.

3. To invite you to consider connecting with a professional loctician like myself to determine if getting help with starting and/or maintaining your locs is the best next step for you.

I've tried to distill and write out the best practices of locs and locking. If you are inclined, you have the information you need to start and maintain your locs.

However, most readers will be best served and have better locking outcomes if they reach out to a professional to see if getting help would make sense.

Anyone interested in locking will gain insights from reading this book. The principles apply whether you are male or female, young or mature. But when writing the book, I had three types of women in mind:

1. Women with wavy, curly, coily, kinky, or

mixed textured hair who want to know which loc method matches their hair texture.

2. Women who are busy professionals who want to know the pros and cons of locking methods for their time constraints and lifestyle.

3. Women who have locs but are looking for information on other maintenance options.

Finally, the Freedom In Locs book was written for the person who agrees with these beliefs:

- Anyone desiring to wear locs is free to do so regardless of race, creed, religion, or background.

- Although locs are essentially matted hair. It is purposefully matted hair. Neglect or uncleanness is not a necessary part of having locs.

- Products can sometimes be helpful but are rarely, if ever, absolutely necessary to achieve a beautiful set of locs.

- Hair is hair. The vast principles that have allowed millions of people in ages past to present to lock their hair are still applicable today.

- It's ok to disagree. We all come to life with different backgrounds and experiences. We can still be friends.

Are we on the same page? Great! This book is for you. I sincerely appreciate you taking the time to continue this journey with me.

My Promise to You

A woman with locs well suited for her hair texture and lifestyle can experience hair liberation and freedom. The information outlined in this book will help you select the loc installation and maintenance method to ensure that you start on the right foot. Or, if you have locs but are not feeling free in your experience, see where you may want to make changes.

Ultimately, by implementing the ideas in this book, you will gain the ability to:

- Have a more carefree relationship with your hair,

Install and maintain your locs if you are so inclined,

- Or have the tools to find someone to help you maintain your locs if you don't want to do it on your own.

Introduction

I get it. I would've liked to have had a book like this specifically for my hair texture in 2001 when I installed my first set of locs.

I didn't know it then, but it would be more than 20 years before I would find the method that works for my lifestyle, temperament, and hair. There would be many false starts and cumulative months of tediously removing sets that weren't quite right.

I have had a love-hate relationship with my hair for as long as I can remember. My hair is thick, and when left to its own devices, it GROWS.

However, the back and sides of my hair are perfectly coily and thick. The top is neither curly nor straight, has tiny rippled waves, and is less dense.

I would not be writing this book if my hair was all one texture. I would probably be a very different person and would not have locs.

Nevertheless, it is. In big and little ways, my fight to find a way to make the two diverse textures make peace has played a more significant part in my life than I'd like to admit.

Why am I sharing this? It has been a long road to get here, and on my 20+ year journey to having a peaceful existence with my hair through locs and locking, I've had to learn a lot. I've had some hair horror stories. I've been taken advantage of, misled, and misinformed.

I have a profound sense of empathy for anyone who just wants to wake up in the morning and go without needing to spend a lot of mental energy worrying about her hair.

What follows is what I:

- Learned in the school of hard knocks,

- Observed over years of doing natural hair as a side hustle,

- Studied during my time in the Natural Hair Care Specialist school.

- Learned through much extracurricular training with various master locticians across the locking and dreading spectrum.

Hopefully, I can save you some of the hassle and heartache I've endured.

Chapter One
Getting Started With Your Why

If you are like most people, the decision to lock your hair isn't something you have come to quickly, and it is most likely a decision that has taken months to years to embrace.

So I'm not going to spend too much time telling you the importance of thinking about the emotional, financial, social, and other costs of starting locs. I'm going to instead have you consider practical lifestyle questions.

Questions to Consider Before Starting

Here are a few questions to think about as you are preparing to get locs:

Are you in the habit of going to the salon, or do you usually DIY? If you go to the salon, have you found a professional to help you along your locking process?

- How often are you accustomed to shampooing your hair?

- Do you currently have any scalp conditions?

- Is your hair currently healthy? If not, is it damaged, dry, or brittle?

- Is your hair short, medium, or long? Are you prepared to see yourself with shorter hair? Are you ready to manage shorter hair? If not, have you factored in the cost of getting extensions?

- What is your lifestyle like? Are you an artist, an athlete, a student, a business professional, or self-employed?

- What hobbies and extracurricular activities

are essential to you? Do you frequent the gym, swim, or work outdoors?

- What look are you ultimately going for? Do you want to make a statement? Or do you just want to simplify your life?

There are no "right" or "wrong" answers. But I would encourage you to grab a notebook and take a moment to write down your answers. As we continue on in the book, you may be more aware of how locking your hair may impact your life based on the answers you give.

Dealing with Family & Friends

You probably already know this, but everyone has their own opinion of locs, locking, and lock wearers. So by extension, they will transfer those opinions to you. This is true even of friends and family who have known you all your life.

Depending on your personality, you may or may not care. But even for the most self-assured, it is hard to face criticism, questioning, and confrontation, especially when it comes from friends and family.

You can "just do it" and let the chips fall where they may. This is easier when you don't have to deal with people who disagree with your decision daily.

You might also consider trying to get some of your loved ones on board or at least gauge the future response by trying out temporary faux locs. It may be easier to deal with thoughtless comments when you haven't invested much time in natural dreads, which is a relatively permanent style.

Reflections to Action

What is your "why"? If you haven't already, write down the answers to the questions above. If your family isn't fully on board, think about how you can have a support system or network in place of loc-friendly people to encourage you as you begin your journey.

Chapter Two

The Best Installation Method for YOU!

When deciding on how to have locs installed and how they will be maintained, it is essential to consider your hair texture, shampoo schedule, and your personal style. When a locking choice is made that aligns with all three elements, most women go on to have an enjoyable relationship with their newly locked hair. When there is a mismatch, there can be a lingering dissatisfaction despite seeming to have what you thought you wanted.

This chapter aims to help you think through these elements to make locking installation and ongoing maintenance decisions that will work best for you for years.

What Are Locs?

Before we look at the various methods of starting locs and how instant locking compares to each, let's first define what a loc is.

Locs or locks are rope-like strands formed by coiling, twisting, braiding, or interlocking hair. Every day, we lose 50 - 100 strands of hair. The shed hair would usually be combed and brushed out but remains in the loc and tangles with the unshed hair.

Routine loc maintenance encourages hair to incorporate into the coiled, twisted, braided, interlocked, or instant-locked hair. Over months or years, the purposeful encouragement of tangling and incorporating creates locs.

Hair Texture & Installation Methods

It was once thought that the only and best method of starting and maintaining locs was with some type of coil or rolling. Today, more and more people of bi-racial and multi-racial ancestry want locs. Locking professionals have had to rethink how locs can be started on hair that will not coil.

This fact has given rise to new methods of starting and maintaining locs, most of which will be explored in this book. Some ways work best with certain hair textures, and others work with most textures of hair to varying degrees. One method works universally to start and maintain locs on any hair texture. Still, it may not be the BEST choice for every situation.

Before we get into that, let's take a quick look at hair texture. There is a wide range of natural ethnic hair textures. They range from soft waves to wavy to curly to tight curls to coily to tight coils to kinky to wiry. Let's take a quick look at each.

- **Soft Waves** - It has a medium wave pattern. It can be fine, to coarse. It is usually of average density. It has limited volume. It is moderately elastic, moves easily, and has a natural shine or sheen.

- **Wavy Hair** - It has a slight wave pattern. It can also range from fine to coarse. Has a higher than average density with moderate volume. It can be moderate to excessively frizzy. Has good elasticity and gentle movement. It is prone to frizzing and tangling. Reflects light with a low shine.

- **Curly Hair** - ranges from large to medium ringlets, spirals, or loops. Ranges from fine to course. It has lots of volume and above-average density. Requires regular moisture. Very elastic. It can be moderate to excessively frizzy and tangly. Reflects light with a low shine.

- **Tight Curls** - Curl formation ranges from medium to tiny ringlets, spirals, or corkscrews. Ranges from fine to coarse. It tangles easily, is frizzy, and is prone to knots at the ends. It is somewhat elastic. It is very dense. Requires daily hydration. It doesn't reflect light and one needs to use oil for shine. **Coily Hair** - This curl configuration can range from small spiral-like curls to tiny ringlets. Hair diameter is fine to coarse. Has lots of volume. It does shrink and is dense. This texture of hair is fragile. It tangles and breaks easily. Requires hydration and oil for shine.

- **Tight Coils** - The hair forms very tight corkscrews or spiral curls. It can range in volume and density. You will have a lot of shrinkage. It is a fragile hair texture prone to tangling at the ends and breakage. This type of hair needs to be repeatedly hydrated with an application of oil for sheen. This texture is often called "spongy."

- **Kinky Hair** - This texture has the smallest of tight curls or coils. It has the most shrinkage when wet. The diameter of the hair strand can be fine to coarse. It is very dense. It is very fragile and very prone to tangling and frizzing. Needs daily hydration and to be oiled often to shine. The texture is often called "cottony."

- **Wiry Hair** - When touched, this texture feels rough or coarse. It may have a zigzag pattern instead of definite curls. The hair diameter can be fine to coarse. It can range in density and volume. It is incredibly fragile and highly prone to tangling and frizzing. Needs intensive hydration and to be oiled often to shine.

Choosing an Installation Method

There are many methods to start locs. Some methods include organic, free form, coils, twists, braids, interlock, and instant locs. We'll only look at the last five methods for installing cultivated locs, and each has pros and cons.

As you think about which method would be best for you, you'll want to keep in mind the following things:

- **Your hair texture** - Is your hair wavy or straight? Is it coarse, tightly curled, or soft?

- **Your hair length** - Is your hair short, medium length, or long?

>   **Your lifestyle** - What types of daily activities do you engage in? Do you exercise or swim regularly? How often do you usually wash your hair?
>
> - **Your personal aesthetic**- How manicured or organic are you comfortable with your hair looking?

As you read the following locking and installation methods, consider your hair texture, length, lifestyle, and personal aesthetic.

Starting Locs with Coils

There are many methods of forming locs that work with the natural coil of your hair. Comb coils, palm rolling, and finger-twisting are all options. Here are some points to remember:

- They are a popular method for starting locs on short to medium hair that is uniformly coily or curly.

- Water soluble gel will help to hold the coils in

place during installation and throughout the locking process.

- Usually produces 60 - 100+ locs ranging from large to small.

- You will need to be careful or wait to wash them as they can come uncoiled when wet. So coils are not ideal for those who need to wash their hair frequently.

- The scalp can be cleansed and freshened between shampoos using the "dry shampoo" method outlined in the chapter on maintenance.

- They will go through a wild, frizzy, and fuzzy stage before reaching full maturity.

- They are usually maintained by retwisting the roots (comb coiling or palm rolling) for consistency.

Coils are a straightforward way to start locking. If your hair doesn't have a consistent curl pattern or you need to shampoo your hair more frequently, the two-strand twist may suit your needs.

Starting Locs with Two-Strand Twists

Starting locks with two-strand twist is straightforward. Once hair is parted for the loc, it is again divided into two sections and then twisted around one's fingers and then around itself to form a rope-like coil of two-plys of hair. Here are some facts about locs that are started with two-strand twists.

- This method is popular for women who have medium to long natural hair.

- Twists are also popular for women with looser curl patterns and mixed textured hair.

- If your hair is thin, this method can give your starter locs the appearance of more volume.

- They have a cylindrical appearance, but the initial twisted sections tend to be fatter/thicker than the coiled or interlocked new growth.

- It can be used to start locs that are very large

(less than 20 locs) to micro-sized (more than 150)

- Twists hold up better to washing and being wet than coils but not as well as braids or instant locs.

- They also can go through a frizzy, fuzzy stage before reaching full maturity, but less so than coils.

- They can be maintained by retwisting the roots (comb coiling or palm rolling) for hair textures that are naturally coily or curly. For looser curl patterns and mixed textured hair, interlocking the new growth is usually the method of choice.

Length and hair texture are usually the elements that lead women to choose to install locs by two-strand twisting their hair.

Starting Locs with Three-Strand Braids

Starting locs with three-strand braids is another widespread method of creating locs. This became the most common alternative way of starting small to tiny to micro-sized locs around the same time that designer locks started with interlocking was coming into prominence.

The process of creating locs with three-strand braids is straightforward. Once hair is parted for the lock. The hair is sectioned again into three sections and braided or plaited. Depending on the hair texture, the hair may be braided almost to the end and then left to naturally coil or curl. Here are some facts about locs that are started with three-strand braids.

- This method is popular for women who have medium to long natural hair.

- Braids are also popular for women with looser curl patterns and mixed textured hair.

- If your hair is very thick, braids can help to control some of the volume.

- Braids hold up best to washing and being wet.

- Generally used to start locs that are medium 80 +/- locs to micro-sized more than 250+

- They can go through a frizzy, fuzzy stage before reaching full maturity, but less so than coils.

- They can have a flattened appearance. This can be helped by finger coiling.

- Sometimes the braiding pattern never goes away. Even after years of having locks, you may have ends of your hair that still show that they were started with braids. For some, this is an aesthetic issue.

- They can be maintained by retwisting the roots (comb coiling or palm rolling) for hair textures that are naturally coily or curly. For looser curl patterns and mixed textured hair, interlocking the new growth is usually the method of choice.

As mentioned before, length and hair texture are usually the elements that lead women to choose to install locs by braiding their hair.

Starting Locs By Interlocking

This method is associated with starting and maintaining very small to micro-sized locs. It involves intertwining the hair from tip to root to create a braid/twist-like pattern in hair. This intertwining can be done with your fingers or with various tools. Although it can be used to start locks of any size, it is most often associated with starting smaller-sized locs.

Interlocking follows a pattern. The pattern is usually related to the face of a clock or the cardinal/ordinal directions. There are many locking patterns or rotations, ranging from 2-point all the way up to 8-points. The most common practice is the 4-point clockwise rotation. That is, the lock is pulled through the base with the following pattern:

- The 4-Point Clockwise Locking Pattern
    - East, South, West, North

- 3 o'clock, 6 o'clock, 9 o'clock, 12 o'clock

- Right to left, up, left to right, down.

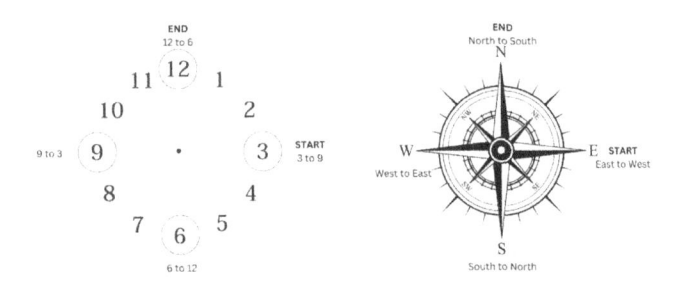

- It is generally accepted best practice to start at 3 o'clock/East/right so that you can end on 12/North/pulling the lockdown.

- It is essential to pay attention to where you are in the rotation so that you don't go through the same point more than once before going to the next point. This can cause holes in the locs. This can lead to weakened locs over time.

- After each rotation, it is important to press down the newly looped/flipped hair toward the tip/base/previously looped/flipped sections of the loc to create a firm hole-free loc.

Interlocking is one of the three methods of starting locs that can also be used for installation and ongoing maintenance (the other two are coils and crocheting/instant locs). Like instant locs, it is a method of creating locked hair using a tool. Here are some facts about locs started by interlocking:

- It is popular for women who have short to medium-length hair.

- Women with looser curl patterns and mixed textured hair also gravitate to interlocking, as mentioned above, for maintenance, if not for installation.

- At first, care may need to be taken when washing interlocked hair to avoid the locs unraveling. This is especially true for looser hair textures.

- Interlocked locs are prone to bunching and slippage if not washed with a care regimen.

- It can be used to start locs that are any size. Most often used to create locs that are small 100+/- locs to micro-sized more than 250+

- They can go through a frizzy, fuzzy stage before reaching full maturity, but it is not as obvious, especially in small sizes.

- They are maintained with interlocking so has a consistent look from root to tip.

- The initial interlocking of long hair is a premium service. But you should not feel pressured to cut your hair if you are willing to pay for it. Or you can opt to have the roots interlocked and the length contained by another method.

- If you have a hard-to-lock hair type, you must take care when washing your hair for the first 6 months to a year. You will need to loosely braid the starter locs into sections and secure those sections with rubber bands before shampooing your hair.

- Like braids, the interlocking pattern may never entirely be obscured in some hair textures. This is more obvious in soft waves to curly and when the locking sizes are large.

Interlocking may not be the first choice for everyone. But interlocking works for ladies with multi-textured hair who want a simple method that looks consistent from beginning to end, is straightforward to maintain and allows for shampoos without worry. This is why this is the method that I chose to install my current set of 150+ small to very small locs.

Starting Instant Locs

Instant Locs, also known as crochet dreadlocks, have been around for quite some time. They were most popular within the straight/ Caucasian/Hispanic/Asian hair-locking community. This is the primary method for creating locs on hair that generally is resistant to forming locs.

Kris McDred can be credited for bringing the concept to prominence within the Afro hair/Traditional locking world with a video he published on youtube on 20 Nov. 2014. That video had received over 10 million views at the time that I was writing this book. Since creating that video, he has created an education program that teaches the instant lock method and various signature locking techniques.

The best way to understand how interlocking is done is to watch that initial video of him performing interlocks that is still available for free on YouTube. That is how I, like many others, first learned the skill several years ago. Or you can enroll in one of his prerecorded video or one-on-one classes and learn from him directly. At the time of the writing of this book, he is still readily available to answer questions and give personalized feedback and support. That's also what I did; it changed how I approached locs. Here are some facts about instant locking:

- Instant locs can start locs on ALL hair types and textures.

- Instant locs can be started on any hair 2" plus up to and beyond bottom length.

- Instant locs look like mature locs from day one, avoiding the months of changes that other locking methods go through before being fully locked.

- Instant locs can be washed from day one.

- Instant locs can be maintained in any way that traditional locs of the same size and texture would be maintained.

- Instant loc maintenance can feel like the scalp is being pinched or pulled, so it may not be the best maintenance method for those with tender heads.

If you want to skip the locking phases, instant locs will take you from loose natural to entirely locked length and look in less than 24 hours.

Loc Method + Hair Texture Chart

Choosing an installation and maintenance method that doesn't match the natural properties of one's hair is just a recipe for frustration. If your hair is mixed-textured, consider using the locking method that works for the *hardest to lock* areas of your hair, over your *entire* head. Here is a chart to give a clearer picture of what we've covered in this chapter:

Before Getting Loc Extensions...

There are several things to consider before getting loc extensions: your hair type, availability of service providers, their installation method, their warranty, and your budget. We'll look at each of these aspects below.

Hair Type

As with any type of extension service, you want to ensure that the hair you have installed matches your hair color and texture. Permanent loc extensions are not an exception.

You want to find an extension provider that uses hair or creates extensions that match your hair type. This is especially true if you have hair that is a soft wave to curly texture. Ideally, your extensions should look like you grew them, not like they were connected to your hair as an afterthought.

Availability of Professionally Trained Service Providers

There has been a sharp rise in cosmetologists, locticians, and natural hair care specialists offering loc extensions. You want to find someone who has taken the time to learn how to execute lock extensions to the highest level. This ensures that you shouldn't have issues with your locs coming out or coming apart in the future.

Their Warranty

When installed correctly, lock extensions shouldn't slip or fall out. A professional instant loc/ crochet dreadlock specialist should be able to confidently stand behind their work. With proper care, high-quality human hair loc extensions can last 1 - 3 years or beyond.

Your Budget

High-quality human hair extensions can cost as much, if not more, than the starter loc installation. Depending on the type of extensions installed and the installation method, there may be a charge to attach them to the ends of your hair. You want to beware of loc extensions whose prices are too good to be true. It is essential to budget for the cost of loc installation, loc extensions/bulk human hair, and attachment when deciding whether to have loc extensions installed.

Methods of Extending Locs

How you extend your starter locs, if you choose to extend them, will generally depend on the method you choose to have the locs installed.

Extending Two-Strand Twists, Three-Strand Braids

You'll continue the installation method with added bulk human hair for twists or braids. Here are principles that are generally followed:

- Starter locs are extended by adding bulk human hair a little at a time until the desired length is achieved.

- It is essential to be careful not to add too much hair towards the end.

- The goal is to extend the natural length while

maintaining the size and amount of hair in the starting twist or plait.

- There shouldn't be any definite lines of demarcation where you can see where the natural hair ended and extension hair was added in.

When the above is done with care by a professional loctician or natural hair care specialist, the look should be seamless. The most important thing with extending starter locs created with twists or braids is getting the bulk human hair that matches. You want a close match to the hair texture and the color on the tips of your hair if it is different from the length.

Extending Interlocked Locs

Since interlocking is a maintenance method as well as an installation method, it should come as no surprise that loc extensions can be added to the end for length. To maintain your hair with interlocking while adding length, interlock the length of your hair to just above the tip. The free hair at the end would be instant locked, and then loc extensions would be added. More information on that process follows.

- Small Width - 0.6cm (80 - 120 locs)

- SMedium Width - 0.8cm (70 - 100 locs)

- Medium Width - 1cm (70 - 80 locs)

- Large Width - 1.2cm (60 - 80 locs)

- XLarge Width - 1.5cm (40 - 50 locs)

How many locs you need will depend on your hair density. If you have average to thick hair, you'll generally have more instant locs installed than those with thin or low-density hair. The parting size that is best for your hair should determine the size of the loc, not the other way around.

For a more natural look, you may consider getting more than one size to account for the varying density of hair throughout our heads. A mix of medium and smedium or smedium and small will look more natural and match the areas of the scalp where locs are smaller/thinner due to less hair (nape, sides, etc.).

Loc Extension Lengths

Commercially made locs are 4" to over 20" inches long. Here are some things to keep in mind when deciding on what length to have installed:

- Four-inch loc extensions are suitable for compensating for the lose of natural length resulting from instant locking of the hair. It will offset the shrinkage and make it seem like you started your locs by just locking your natural hair.

- Six-inch loc extensions will give short locs more styling options and look like a layered haircut when installed on very short instant locs.

- Eight-inch loc extensions allow for ponytails as well as shoulder-length curls.

- Ten to twenty-plus inch loc extensions are good for those who are used to wearing very long hair.

When deciding the length to get, remember that the extension will be installed at THE TIP of the instant loc. You will lose two to three inches of length with the instant loc installation. As mentioned above, four inches will offset that loss. Everything else is extra.

Loc Extension Colors

Commercially made human hair locs extensions come in the standard color such as 1b, 2, 3, 5, 5, 6, 8, 12, 24, 22, 613, 33, 32, 31, 27, 33D as well as novelty colors and ombre blends.

When deciding what color to choose, you'll want to select the color that best matches the color of the hair at your ends.

Handcrafted Premade Human Hair Lock Extensions

Your hair texture doesn't match commercially made human hair loc extensions. This happens. You may need to consider seeking a specialty permanent human hair loc extension creator. You want to find someone who specializes in crafting locs in your hair type. The loctician installing your locs may offer this service, especially if they are accustomed to working on all hair types.

You can expect to pay more for the loc extension creation than the instant loc installation. This is because the loctician will need to purchase human hair to match your hair and create the permanent loc extensions to be installed. Generally, you'll be asked to leave a deposit to cover the cost of purchasing the hair and making the loc extension before your installation.

Installing Permanent Loc Extensions

Permanent loc extensions are definitely an investment, so you want to ensure that you get the best life out of the investment by ensuring that they are correctly installed. The method by which your loc extensions are installed, will make a difference between whether or not your loc extensions look real or like extensions.

Seamless Crochet Attachment of Premade Permanent Loc Extensions

The benchmark method for installing premade permanent loc extensions on any hair type, be it bone

Reflection to Action

What, if anything, do you need to do to prepare your hair for loc installation?

Chapter Five

Getting Your Sections Sorted

The section size and layout of your locs will make a big difference in the overall look of your locs. So how big should you make the sections for your locs? The density of your hair will help to determine that.

Here are some things to consider:

- The average part sizing for naturally textured hair is about 1" x 1", which works out to about 60 - 70 locs.

- Thicker hair can accommodate smaller section

sizes (less than 3/4" to 1/2") and more locs (80 to well over 100 locs.)

- Thinner hair should be parted slightly larger than 1" x 1" and will have fewer locs (usually less than 60)

- Small to micro-sized locs range from 1/3" to ¼."

Aside from density, you will want to think about your lifestyle.

- The more locs you have, the more maintenance you'll need to do or have done.

- Thin locs can quickly merge if you don't stay on top of separating them at their bases to keep them from joining together.

- Thin locs often take longer to mature.

- Thicker locks can take a bit longer to dry. Something to consider if you swim or exercise a lot.

Those are just a few things that might make you choose one size over another.

Parting Size Versus Eventual Loc Size

One of the reasons to consider getting a professional loctician who understands the locking process is that they understand this fundamental parting principle:

- The size of the initial parts is more important than the compressed size of the initial hair.

- When locs are first installed, the hair is generally compressed. As the hair grows, falls out, and is intermeshed together, the loc begins to grow and expand. Mature locs are typically two to three times larger than the initial loc.

Remember to part your hair understanding your locs will expand. If you don't, you may be unhappy with the size of your locks.

Micro-sized Isn't Necessarily the Best

I feel more people err on the side of too small than on the side of too large when thinking of what sized small locs to install. If you:

- don't enjoy doing your hair and
- don't have access to someone who can consistently help you keep your locks maintained,
- don't have a backup if that person is unavailable,

I would encourage you not to opt for the smallest lock sizes.

Remember, micro-sized locs are as much of a lifestyle as a hairstyle, and you want to ensure that the size you choose adds to your quality of life and doesn't subtract from it.

Loc Parting Styles

After you've decided on the size of your locs, you may want to think about how you want them arranged on your head. This is determined by the style or shape that they are parted in. The following are some common parting styles:

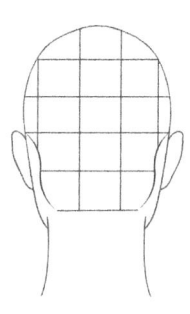

Grid - sections are arranged like grid paper. Very spacey - shows lots of your scalp. Works for thick hair and/or small dread sizes. Useful for styling that requires clean parting.

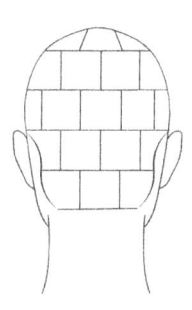

Bricklay - Sections staggered so that the verticle lines are directly above the middle of the lock on the row below it. Good scalp coverage and works with any hair type.

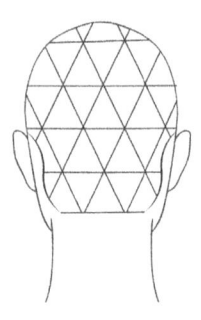

Triangle - Created by creating horizontal rows and dividing the sections with alternating diagonal partings. Good scalp coverage but is more tricky than brick.

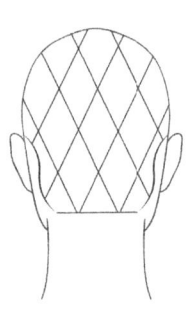

Diamond - Sections are created by making diagonal lines across the scalp. Dreads fall between dreads on the rows below. Most challenging pattern to execute.

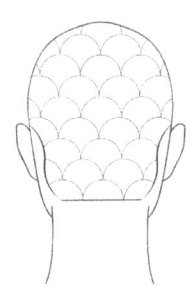

Fan/Half-moon/Crescent/Fish Scales - are similar to bricklaying in that the bottom of the subsequent locks are in the middle of the locks below it. Excellent scalp coverage and gives a structured organic look.

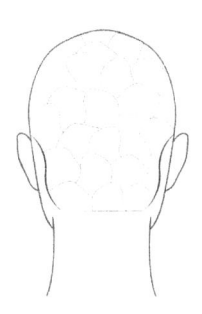

Grab and Go/Organic - Sections are grabbed with less effort to make the locks a particular shape while keeping sizing relatively the same.

The parting will depend on what you feel comfortable executing or your loctician offers.

Professional Parting Help is Worth It

The previous information is a lot to take into consideration. And I know the feeling (and the relief) that comes from letting someone else figure it out and happily sitting in the salon chair.

Parting is so important to the locking process and the foundation of your locks that it is something that you want to have done by someone who can do it so that you don't second guess later on.

If you cannot get to a loctician and plan to DIY, you might consider getting a local braider to part your hair.

Just put the braids in the size you want your locs to be. Yes, you will take them out, but you will get better service and results if you let them create a style that will look nice when they are done. They can take a picture of you for their portfolio.

You don't need to explain why you want them and what you plan to do. In fact, it is probably best not to talk about it. Seriously. Not helpful. Why? Because you may confuse them as to what you want.

Check portfolios before calling around. You want someone who creates neat, consistent sections/parts. You will probably get bricklaying parts. If you want some other types, make sure it is something that they do regularly by looking at their portfolio.

What you will do is take down each individual braid and create your loc using your chosen loc installation method.

Consider Getting a Friend to Help You

No local braiders? No problem. Ask a friend to help you. Seriously, going it alone is so not fun.

If you like to DIY, this is the part, even more so than locking, where you might want to think about getting help. In theory, you just draw lines across your scalp with a comb. In practice, you want those lines and sections to be even and relatively consistent. That is way more challenging than you might suspect.

I have had to part my hair for various styles, including installing my own sets of locs. On every occasion, somewhere along the line, I would think. I wish I had someone to help me. EVERY. SINGLE. TIME.

The second pair of eyes and hands can give you peace of mind. It will also cut the process in half as you are not having to consult mirrors and contort your body to get your parts right.

The simplest thing is to let them section and rubber band section or twist your whole head. If anything needs to be tweaked later, you can do that after they've done the most challenging part for you.

How to See the Back Of Your Head

No pro, friend, or family to help you? I hear you. I've been there. This is the method I used to install 350 micro-sized locks with precise grid sectioning on myself. It was a grind. But it worked so well that people thought they were done by someone else.

It really wasn't a complicated setup. Here's what you will need:

- Your phone

- Screen mirroring app for your phone

- Way to position the phone behind your head. (Arkon mount, selfie stick, etc.)

- A computer or tablet

- Wifi

You'll download the app on your phone and open it. It will give you an address to put into a browser's address bar. Put that into the tablet or computer, which should be facing you.

Click "Start Mirroring" on your phone. Refresh the page on your computer and/or tablet. You should see whatever is on your phone screen. Navigate to your camera and open the photo like you were going to take a picture. Now position the phone so that it is behind your head, pointing to the area you need to see.

Walah! You have eyes on the back of your head.

You're welcome!

Reflection to Action

What size and parting shape are you leaning towards for your locs?

Chapter Six

The Professional Loc Installation

Getting your locs installed can be a liberating time! This chapter will look at an overview of what you can expect if you get them professionally done.

The Consultation

During your initial new client consultation, the two of you will talk to ensure that you are on the same page.

This is an excellent opportunity for you to get any questions you may have about the process answered.

There may be a fee for the consultation. Sometimes that will go towards the cost of your installation, and sometimes it is a separate service.

When everything is done, you will probably be asked to put down a portion of the estimated cost of installation to book the date. If you are ordering extensions, you will generally be asked to pay for those up front if they are custom-made.

Once those things are taken care of, and the date is on the calendar, you're set!

You will want to be aware of the cancelation policy. Things happen, and canceling might be unavoidable. You will want to know how much notice is needed to cancel/change the date and how funds already paid will be handled.

The Lead-Up

During the consultation, they will likely tell you how they would have you prepare for the installation and what products they recommend. You'll want to take notes of these instructions and follow them to have the best installation experience.

What to Bring & What Not to Bring

As you think about what to pack, remember you'll be sitting for long periods. So bring something so that you'll be comfortable. Ensure your digital devices are charged and have the cords and blocks you need. They may have water and snacks, but it isn't a bad idea to bring some of your own, especially if you have special dietary needs.

They may stop to let you both take lunch or work straight through and have you eat in the chair. If the salon isn't close to places that deliver, it might be a good idea to pack lunch. This is an excellent question to ask during the consultation.

Projects and hobbies that can be done on your lap if that is your type of thing can also be good.

Do you have low pain tolerance? You may want to consider taking some pain medication if you will have instant locs done before the service starts and at the proper interval during and after.

Of course, bring a positive, happy attitude!

What not to bring is as important as what to bring, or at least ask before bringing.

- Children - it isn't a good idea to bring kids unless your loctician explicitly says it is ok. The exception is for a baby that will be content being held on your lap.

- Extra people - unless it is stated on their website that you are welcome to bring a friend, don't assume it is ok.

- A bad attitude. We feed off of each other. You want the environment that you are starting off in to be good. Feed that with good energy.

After Locking Care

Your locks are in! Now what? Your loctician will have their own aftercare instructions for you. Which may include their recommended products which they may carry.

You may also need to "settle into" your new look. The euphoria that is present at your installation may wane. Especially if you get grief from family and friends about your decision.

You'll want to take care of your own mental health. Have a supportive group of people who appreciate the beauty of locs or seek some out before your installation. They will be able to encourage you on days when your locs aren't doing or looking quite like you hope.

It is not uncommon to experience a bit of "buyer's remorse" a few days or even weeks after getting your installation. Did you make the right decisions? Should your locks be smaller (or bigger)? Is too much scalp showing? All the things.

It's ok.

It can happen when you make a choice that isn't easily undone. It will pass. Remember why you decided to get locs. And having some pretty scarves and head wraps on hand can help too! It is amazing how a scarf around the hairline can change the look!

You made a good decision, and you didn't make it lightly. You'll look back and wonder why you didn't do it sooner. I promise.

Reflection to Action

After reading this chapter, what questions might you want to discuss with a loctician before your installation? How do you feel about the process? As you picture yourself going through the process, what would you need to do to ensure you have the best experience possible?

Chapter Seven

Maintenance: Taking Care of Your Investment

Although locs can be very low-maintenance, if you want locs that turn heads in a good way, you'll need to invest a little time in regular maintenance. The basic maintenance regimen for locked hair is very simple, and it consists of two main things:

- Keep your locs clean

- Keep your locs separated.

It is that simple. Everything we'll be looking at in the rest of this chapter falls in one or the other of these maintenance categories.

Products, Products, Products

One of the nicest things about having locs is the fact that your product usage can come way down. For those of us who were never product junkies, to begin with, that is good news. We don't have to start!

Do you struggle with always wanting to get that miracle thing that will make the miracle claim? This section is mainly for you, to give you permission to trust that left to its devices, your hair will lock. Adding products to speed up the process in the short term will only lead to problems in the long term.

What goes on your locs needs to easily come out. Remember this is the principle when considering what to put on your locs. You want to use water-soluble products that easily rinse away with water.

The reason is that whatever doesn't rinse out of your locs doesn't make them stronger. It contributes to build-up. And build-up is the beginning of death to long-term healthy locking dreams.

Best Practices for Washing

So how do we avoid build-up from any products and the natural oils in our hair? By regularly shampooing our locs.

How often you shampoo will depend on a variety of things, including. The loc installation method, the age of your locs, your lifestyle, and your working environment.

It is generally accepted that twice weekly is on the high-frequency end of how often one should wash their locs, and once a month is on the low frequency. Starting when your locs are new, you want to wash your locks at least once a week. It is a hideous myth that dirty hair locs best. Nothing could be further from the truth.

Shampoo

When choosing a shampoo, you want to select something that is sulfate, parabens, dye, and residue free.

Each loctician has favorites and ones they don't recommend for various reasons.

No matter what shampoo you choose, the following practices will help you get the most out of your wash and avoid inadvertently having shampoo build-up in your locks.

- Dilute your shampoo - You can do this in an applicator bottle. Which makes it easier to

- Focus on your scalp - that is mainly where the oils and dead scalp cells are.

- Let the residual suds cleanse your locs- unless you work in a dirty job where your locs get dirty, you shouldn't need to put globs of shampoo directly on your locks.

- Test your water - the minerals in hard water reacting with shampoo can lead to build-up. Hard water is also hard to lather, leading to more product usage and build-up.

- If you have hard water, do an apple cider vinegar (ACV) and rinse every other shampoo.

Generally, cream-based or thick conditioners aren't used because they leave residue on the locs. They are hard to rinse entirely out of locs, which can lead to build-up, which leads to mold and odor.

"Dry" Shampoo/ Scalp Refresher

You may be in a situation where you cannot wash your locs on your regular schedule. Maybe you just want/need to do a scalp refresher between your regular shampoo. In those cases, you can cleanse your scalp without wetting your hair.

The basics of what you need are:

- Gauze, cheesecloth, or lint-free cotton towel
- Astringent - Witch Hazel/ Seabreeze

As always, I would suggest that you work methodically from back to front to ensure that you thoroughly clean all the areas of your scalp. Here is what you would do:

- Apply astringent to the cloth and rub the part/separation line on your scalp.

If you have new growth/loose hair, you can rub the area of the scalp under the loc.

- Change out cloths or move to a clean area as it is soiled.

The nice thing about doing a dry shampoo/ scalp refresh is that it provides cleaning with light scalp stimulation. Overall, it's really good.

Again, this isn't a long-term substitute for regular washing, just a tool to have in your kit if the need arises.

Suggestions for Separating

Separating your locs is best done after washing your locs when the hair is still damp but not wet. There are a variety of methods that can be used to separate your locks, sometimes called cracking or popping your locks. They generally involve pulling locks apart from tip to root.

The following method is methodical. It will ensure that you maintain your parts, address all the locs on your head without accidentally missing any, and have the least unnecessary breakage.

- You will be working from back to front. Secure your locs in a high ponytail if you have lots of hair. You can also use clips.

- Use your fingers to carefully separate the very bottom horizontal row of locs.

- Work along the original parting lines pulling from ROOT to TIP.

- Smooth any hair that doesn't belong in the bottom row up towards the next row.

- Once you have the bottom row separated, carefully separate the VERTICAL part lines

- Repeat on the next row. Progressively working up.

Best Practices for Drying

Making sure your hair gets dry between shampoos or periods of being wet is super important to avoid mold and mildew in your locs. Here are some simple things that you can do to ensure that your hair is dry:

- Wash your hair early in your day to avoid sleeping on wet locs.

- Get a microfiber towel to help with drying if your locks are thick or your hair has a tendency to hold water.

- Let your hair hang loose and unbound to allow air to circulate between your locks.

- If you don't have hours to let your locks air dry, use a blow dryer or bonnet dryer to speed up the process.

- Schedule your shampoo day(s) so you are not in a rush.

- Wear a shower cap when you are showering.

- Wear a swim cap when swimming.

Here are a few things to avoid:

- Avoid pulling your wet/damp locks into a ponytail, braids, or buns.

Avoid wearing caps, hats, or headwraps if your locs are damp.

- Avoid washing your hair before bed.

Sometimes we can't help having our locs wet for longer than we would like, getting caught in torrential rain storms in the summer without an umbrella, for example. But those types of things are few and far between.

Afro-Kinky Hair Root Maintenance Methods

The lovely thing about instant locs in afro-textured hair is that, for the most part, there are a variety of options by which you can maintain your new growth. You can:

- Palm Roll/Loc Smyth Retwist

- Comb Retwist

- Interlock

- Crochet Maintenence/ Crochet Retwist

The first two options are offered at most traditional loc salons. Interlocking is becoming more and more widely available. And whoever installed your instant locs will most likely be able to maintain the new growth with retwisting if you so choose.

When deciding what maintenance method you would like to use, you want to remember the pros and cons of each. Select a strategy that will work the best with your lifestyle and hairstyle.

Interlocking too tightly and too often can lead to traction alopecia, hair loss caused by excessive and prolonged tightness at your roots. You generally want to wait 6 - 8 weeks between retightening sessions. If you need to neaten up your look for a special occasion, consider having a retwist done. It will temporarily freshen up your locs until you get your scheduled service.

For locs tightened by retwisting, it is a good idea to ensure that the locs are always twisted in the same direction.

Straight, Wavy, or Mixed Textured Hair

If you have a harder-to-lock hair type or mixed textured hair, you will have fewer maintenance options, but options nonetheless!

- Interlocking

- Crochet Maintenenc/ Crochet Retwist

If your hair is loosely curly or mixed-textured with a good bit of curly or coily areas, then interlocking may be a good choice. The curly coily areas may match the instant loc portion of your hair, so the interlocking may become less evident over time. The straighter sections may never completely lose the patterned braided look. The smaller the locs, the less noticeable this is.

If you are thinking that you might at some point want to maintain your hair yourself, between interlocking and crochet maintenance interlocking, with training is easier to do.

The other option is to crochet or have your new growth crocheted. I look at how to care for and maintain locs in straight to wavy hair in my book *Dreadful*

Beauty, which can be found at www.dreadfulbeauty.com.

As mentioned above, the person who installed your instant locs will likely be able to provide this service for you.

The cost of Maintenence

When it comes to what you'll expect to pay. The cost of maintenance, from least expensive to most, would be:

- Retwist

- Interlock

- Crochet

This is because of the supply and demand and the increased skill level each method takes to do it correctly. How much you will pay per maintenance session will depend on:

- the number of locs you have,

- the length of time you've gone between maintenance sessions,

- and whether or not you have any repair work that needs to be done.

Coloring Your Locs

Coloring your locs is best left to a professional. That is a cosmetologist with a successful track record in coloring locs. It isn't something you want to attempt to do yourself because if done wrong, you can do irreparable damage to your locs.

This is because, unlike with loose natural hair, it is very, very, very hard to thoroughly rinse all of the chemicals for coloring your locs out. They will continue working and over-processing your hair if they are not rinsed out properly. This can lead to weakening and damaged locks down the line.

A cosmetologist who understands coloring locs will know that only the outside of the body of the locs needs to be colored. There is no need to work the color inside the locs. Someone who doesn't deal with locs might not realize this.

There are different ways to change the color of your locs. Going darker is usually better than lightening your hair. Semi-permanent dyes are generally better than permanent ones. And bleaching your locs should be avoided.

Covering Your Locs

Wraps, scarves, and bandanas serve an efficient purpose in your loc-wearing life. They can protect your hair from dust, debris, and damage from snags when worn during certain activities.

Prevention is better than cure in the battle to keep random junk from embedding in your locks. Here are some situations where you might want to consider covering your locs:

- Working in dusty environments, cleaning, construction, or aggressive gardening.

- Baking

- Painting overhead

Walking through areas where your hair might get snagged, in the woods

Now, if you are cool with how the above might add character to your locs, that is fine too!

Swimming with Locs

If you love to swim, you'll be happy to know that having locs will not put a stop to a favorite pastime. Depending on the type of water, swimming can be beneficial to the progress of your locking process.

You'll want to keep some principles in mind if you like to spend a lot of time in the water.

- Locs do best when not left wet/damp for long periods, more than 5 - 6 hours.

- Plan to thoroughly dry your hair between times in the water.

- A bonnet dryer will help.

- Saltwater can be helpful in the locking process. But you don't want to overdo it.

- Chlorine should be rinsed out as you would with loose natural hair, but it is generally not detrimental.

- Freshwater, ponds, lakes, creeks, and rivers have microorganisms that can reside in your locks. It is best to do a detox after swimming in fresh water.

Due to the popularity of locs, a wide variety of swimming caps sized for locs can be found and purchased online. You may want to consider getting one if you swim regularly.

Reflection to Action

Is there anything that you might need to consider getting to prepare for having locs? What are they? Take a moment and write down anything that you might want to have on hand after your installation to ensure a good transition into your new locked life.

Chapter Eight

Recipes for Healthy Dreads

Herbs and oils provide a fantastic alternative to the usage of commercially made products. Many companies that cater to loc wearers create products from all-natural sources.

Are you into or interested in using common herbs, essential oils, vegetable oils, and natural botanicals? This chapter will give you additional resources you can use with your locs.

Although many of these herbs and oils can be ingested, this chapter is only covering the external application of them. Before applying any natural product, you should consider doing a patch test. And, of course, avoid anything to which you may be allergic.

Conditioning with Natural Oils

You may find that your locs feel dry and brittle. This is because the natural oils from your scalp are unable to travel down the length of your hair as they would if your hair were not in locs but in a loose natural state.

The solution is to use light natural oils as needed to supply the absence of the oils created by your scalp. When looking for an oil to use, you want to find something fast absorbing and liquid at room temperature.

No more than a thimble is needed for your entire head. Oil is best applied after shampooing while the hair is damp but not wet.

Some carrier oils that fit the bill are:

- **Apricot Seed Oil** - Softens dry hair
- **Avocado Oil** - Stimulates growth & restores dehydrated/damaged hair.

- **Fractionated Coconut Oil** - Regenerative, helps brittle hair.

- **Grapeseed Oil** - Moisturizes dry, brittle hair. Strengthens hair cuticle.

- **Sweet Almond Oil** - Reduces itching and inflammation.

Herbs and Essential Oils

Herbs and essential oils can also be valuable to your maintenance schedule. Essential oils are best added to recipes at a 5% - 10% ratio because of their inherent natural potency.

Many beneficial herbs are used in herbal rinses and in hair oil forms. Here are a few commonly used with locs and their benefits.

- **Peppermint** - Oily scalp, Anti-Dandruff, Astringent

- **Lavender** - Hair growth, cell rejuvenation, softener, conditioner, astringent

- **Rosemary** - Oily scalp, hair loss, hair growth, anti-dandruff, softener, conditioner, astringent

- **Tea tree** - Antiseptic, anti-dandruff, astringent

- **Lemon (juice)** - antiseptic, astringent

- **Eucalyptus** - Oily scalp, antiseptic, scalp soother, anti-dandruff,

- **Sage - Antiseptic, hair loss, hair growth, scalp soothers, anti-dandruff, conditioner, astringent.**

- **Basil** - Oily scalp, moisturizer, hair growth

- **Thyme** - Oily scalp, antiseptic, hair loss, hair growth, conditioner.

- **Chamomile** - Antiseptic, moisturizer, scalp soother, astringent

Natural Hair Lightening & Coloring

Herbs and the juices of fruits and plants have been used for millennia for dying. If you want a bit of a gradual change, the following recipes with a little time and sun can provide that.

Dark Coffee Hair Dye - Brew 2 - 3 cups of dark roast coffee double strength. Let cool. Use a bowl or basin to catch liquid saturate locs until completely covered. Cover with a plastic bag and let sit for 1 hour. Rinse with cool water.

Lemon Juice Chamomile Hair Lightener - Add the juice of 1 lemon and a cup of double-brewed chamomile tea to a spray bottle. Spray on your hair and go out in the sun for 30 minutes. Lightning effects will depend on your hair's natural color.

Acid Rinses

Our hair/scalp's natural pH ranges from 4.5 to 5.5 on the pH scale, which is slightly acidic. Distilled water is 7, which is neutral, and ammonia is around 12.

Acid rinses can help to restore the hair's natural pH balance. They are also helpful in removing residual soap and debris from locs.

Here is how to make an acid rinse. Any of the following ingredients can be mixed with water at a ratio of 95:5. That is, 95% water to 5% acid.

- Citric acids - lemon juice, lime juice, orange juice, grapefruit juice, cactus juice.

- Apple Cider Vinegar or Distilled Vinegar

- Tartaric Acid - wine, champagne, beer (leave odors must be rinsed out)

Herbal Rinses & Refreshing Sprays

Herbal rinses are a natural residue-free way to condition and nourish your locs. They can help address issues you may have with your scalp or locs. Or they can be used cosmetically to enhance color or add fragrance.

The primary method for creating and using a herbal infusion for a rinse or spray is as follows:

Mix herbs to be used in a bowl or french press

- Boil water and pour over herbs
- Let steep for 20 - 30 minutes or longer.
- Strain and add in cool water as needed if still hot.
- Pour into a bottle and add in any essential oils and shake.

The mixture can be used as the final rinse after shampooing, or it can be poured into a spray bottle, lightly sprayed on the scalp, and locs daily. Store in the fridge for up to a week.

Chapter Nine

WHEN THINGS GO WRONG

I wish I could tell you that having locs is all sunshine and rainbows. Sometimes it is. But more often, there are hiccups along the way.

The good news is that there is usually a solution for most problems that you will encounter as you go along your locking journey.

Dissatisfaction with Your Locs

How to deal with this will totally depend on when this occurs in your locking journey. If it is early on, as I mentioned above, it may be natural "buyer's remorse." This is especially true if you had your locks done by a professional loctician whose work you admire. It will pass.

If that isn't the case, try to figure out what is bothering you about your locks. Is it:

- The sizing

- The parting

- The way that the locs look/feel

- The length

How the locs look and feel might be able to be fixed with crocheting. Length can be added. If the locs are too small, you may be able to combine them without needing to start over.

If you hate the parts or feel they are too thick/big. You may need to remove them and start over again. But don't worry, it can be done, and if your locs are less than a year old, it should be pretty straightforward. More on loc removal is below.

Thinning/Weak Locs

What to do about thinning locs will depend on where they are thinning. At the roots, it could be over-maintenance, hormonal changes (pregnancy, medication, age-related), or heavy extensions.

Thinning along the lock's length can come from improper maintenance methods/sessions, wearing tight beads, bands, or wraps.

Once you determine what is causing the problem, it is easier to know how to fix it. If possible, stop or correct what caused it. The actual thin or weak spots along the locs can be rectified with crochet maintenance.

Mold in Your Locs

This is one of those issues where prevention is better than cure. You want to avoid keeping your locs damp for extended periods.

Once mold is in your locs, evidenced by having locks that have a dank, musty odor similar to that of a wet towel. Then the job is to kill the mold.

Due to the nature of locs, even after the mold is dead, it is hard, if not impossible, to totally remove it from the inside of your lock.

Super Skinny Locs

If you feel that your locks are too small, you don't necessarily need to start over. It is possible to combine locks using crochet repair techniques. When done correctly, you cannot distinguish combined locs from natural locs of the same size.

Again prevention is better than cure. To avoid locs that are too small for your hair or lifestyle, check out the earlier chapter on parting above.

Loopy Bumpy Locs

This isn't always a bad thing. Some people like locs that have a little bit more "character." But if your loops and bumps steal the show, they can generally be fixed with crochet maintenance. The age of your locs will determine the extent to which you'll totally remove them.

Frizzy Locks

This is kinda par for the course. The frizz will go away, at least that frizz along the body of the locs, as your locks mature. Palm rolling after washing can help, especially when your locks are new.

Avoid the temptation of putting tons of products on your locs in an attempt to "keep the frizz down." What goes on needs to come off sometime. And you will actually start a vicious cycle of scrubbing your locs to remove the product that will make them frizz more and then putting more product to keep down the frizz.

Products lead to build-up, which can contribute to mold. Not good.

And DO NOT trim the frizz with scissors. Doing so can affect the integrity of your locs over time as you accidentally cut the hairs that form the mesh that makes up your locs. Just resist the temptation.

All locks are a bit frizzy at times. It's ok. It is just a part of being a loc wearer.

Uneven Locs

If you have locs of different lengths and want them a little more consistent, loc extensions are a good option.

Or, if you are ready for a change, you can always have your locs cut to make them more even.

Removing Locs

Yes, locs can be removed without cutting off all of your hair, and I've done it with my own sets. Once on 60+, almost 3-year-old locks, and again on 350+ 6-month-old locks.

It isn't quick or easy, but it can be done. It will usually take 2 - 3 times longer to take them out than put them in, especially if they are mature.

The oldest areas, those closest to the ends, will be the most challenging to remove. You may want to consider trimming/cutting a few inches off to make the take down a little easier if your locks are very mature and long.

Some people's hair reacts better to being unraveled dry, while others need heavy use of conditioner to get the locs out. ONE METHOD DOESN'T FIT ALL. It is worth doing some test loc removal before dumping the bottle of conditioner on your head.

Some oils work better than a conditioner or detangling completely dry.

A helpful tool to help with removal can be found in the craft section with the loom knitting supplies. It is a loom knitting tool. It works like the end of a rat tail comb, but it is easier to hold and use.

Chapter Ten

How We Help People Get Beautiful Locs

I hope by now you can see how starting your locs on the right foundations and proper ongoing maintenance can lead you to have a beautiful head of locs..

Choosing the right partner to help you start or maintain your locs can be challenging. Professional locticians skilled in a variety of locking methods and able to cater to any hair are few and far between. It is tempting to throw your hands up in the air and let anyone do your hair or do your best to DIY when you'd rather not.

It is worth seeking out a professional loctician. Doing so can help you have a better start to your locking journey or get you on the right track if your locs started out less than ideal.

We Give Educated Guidance

Many professional locticians have completed specialized training to hone their skills in this craft. Some have apprenticed with other master locticians. Others have taken on and offline courses. Others have brought their background in formal hair education to their work with locs..

For many of us, this is the focus of our business. So we are invested in being our best and providing the guidance and education to help our clients have the best locking experience possible.

We Share Informed Suggestions

It is one thing to google, "what to do when _____." It is another thing to have a professional look at your locs, understand your background, goals, and lifestyle, and give suggestions specific to your situation.

There are few one-size-fits-all answers. And what may work for someone else whose hair may resemble yours may not work best for you.

Everyone is different. We consider those differences when seeking to provide you with an experience tailored for you and your locs..

We Provide Empathetic Support

Most locticians have or have had locs of some type at some point in their lives. Our own locking journeys may have been the spark for our decision to provide the service to others.

So we can empathize with you. We get it because we've been through it ourselves and have also helped others.

Chapter Eleven

The Next Step

Congratulations! You are one step closer to hair freedom through locs. I hope I have opened your eyes to the possibilities of starting locs in a way that works for you. And hopefully, you are excited about the potential of working with me or another professional multi-textured hair locking specialist to get your locs started.

Think about the satisfaction you'll get when someone tells you, "I love your locs! They are so beautiful!"

Feel the joy of waking up and going without needing to give a second thought to what you need to do to your hair.

Trust me, it is gratifying and will make you wonder why you didn't make the decision to loc your hair sooner.

Don't Lose Your Momentum

As I mentioned earlier in the book, I wrote it for two primary reasons:

1. to help, inspire and motivate readers like you;

2. to extend an invitation to see if getting professional help with locking your hair makes sense - for both all parties involved..

Let me ask you to consider these three questions and answer them in your mind.

1. Would having locs installed help to simplify your hair care regime?

2. Are you ready to commit to having your hair loc to gain freedom from loose natural hair stress?

3. Do you value working with an expert to start

your locking journey, guide you along the path to bring out the best in your hair, and help you prevent mishaps and mistakes?

If your answers are three yeses, then you really have three pathways in front of you at this very moment.

1. You can close this book and do nothing with the information I shared. (If you have gotten this far, I sure hope this isn't an option ;-))

2. You can start your locs yourself - on your own- by leveraging the tips, tactics, and strategies I have just given you.

3. You can ensure that your locs or locs and extensions are started off on a solid foundation by scheduling a Loc Consultation Call to discuss your hair locking goals.

If you are serious about having locs that look good and that last, you have nothing to lose by choosing the third pathway.

This call holds the key to unlocking the freedom of having professionally crafted locs and extensions if desired.

The rest of this chapter is about how to schedule a call with me, but I am only one person. It is a possibility that I may not have availability when you reach out. That is why I network with other locking professionals to whom I can refer. So no matter if you are down the street or across the country, feel free to book a call. If I can't help you, I will refer you to a loctician who can.

How to Schedule Our Call

Would you like to schedule a call to speak with me about starting your locs? Here's what to do:

1. Visit OOAKandBespoke.com

2. Click and click on the"Let's Chat" button in the upper right hand corner of the website. Alternatively, you can email me at ooakandbespoke@gmail.com!

I look forward to hearing from you and, more importantly, working together to start your locking journey with a one-of-a-kind and bespoke set of locs.

Thank you!

Amy McKnight,
Licensed Natural Hair Care Specialist
Loctician/Owner
OOAK & Bespoke Natural Hair Salon

Bibliography

Bailey, Diane Carol. *Milady Standard Natural Hair Care & Braiding*. Milady, a Part of Cengage Learning, 2014."Which Length Should I Choose for My Loc Extensions?" *Mukisa Locs | Loc Extensions*, https://mukisalocs.com/blogs/news/which-length-should-i-choose-for-my-loc-extensions.

Bilal-Ali, Aishah. "Loctician Certification Online School." *Natural Hair Class*, https://www.naturalhairclass.com/bundles/loctician-certification.

Bonner, Lonnice Brittenum. *Nice Dreads: Hair Care Basics and Inspiration for Colored Girls Who've Considered Locking Their Hair*. Three Rivers Press, 2005.

Evans, Nekena. *Hairlocking: Everything You Need to Know African, Dread & Nubian Locks*. Eworld Inc, 2010.

Fleming , JoAnna. *LIFE LESSONS & LOCS: Loose Natural Hair Confessions & Loc Maintenance Lessons*. JoAnna Fleming, 2020.

George, M. Michele. *The Knotty Truth: Creating Beautiful Locks on a Dime!: A Comprehensive Guide to Creating Locks*. Manifest Publishing Enterprises, 2010.

"Kris McDred Loctician." *Kris McDred*, 26 Apr. 2022, https://krismcdred.com/kris-mcdred-loctician/.

Liong-A-Kong, Mireille. *Going Natural How to Fall in Love with Nappy Hair*. Sabi Wiri, 2004.

Making Dreadlocks Using a Tool. Nappylocs, 2015.

"Dreadlocks." *Wikipedia*, Wikimedia Foundation, 23 Aug. 2022, https://en.wikipedia.org/wiki/Dreadlocks.

"FAQs." *Legacy Locs*, https://legacylocs.com/pages/faqs.

King, Cherie M. "5 Questions You Should Ask Your New Loctician." *Dr Locs*, https://drlocs.com/blogs/articles/5-questions-you-should-ask-your-new-loctician.

King, Cherie M. "What Is the Best Way to Start Locs?" *Going Natural*, 7 May 2019, https://going-natural.com/what-is-the-best-way-to-start-locs/.

McDred, Kris. "Instant Dreadlocks." *YouTube*, YouTube, 20 Nov. 2014, https://www.youtube.com/watch?v=VXfPvBw1Q8Y.

"Need to Know: The Difference between Locs and Dreadlocks." *Instant Arẹ̀wà Hair*, https://www.instantarewahair.com/blogs/news/need-to-know-the-difference-between-locs-and-dreadlocks.

Acknowledgments

This book wouldn't be possible if it were not for many people's support, encouragement, and inspiration.

To my husband, Conrad McKnight, my daughter Amelia McKnight, my mom Rose Knight and my brother Phil Knight when I have a project, I'm like a dog with a bone. Thank you for checking in, helping out, listening, and being patient with me as I finished this.

To Ms. Latonya Evans, owner/director of the Millinemum Trade Academy, thanks for working with my schedule so that I could complete the program and get legal ;-).

FREEDOM IN LOCS

To all the Millinemum Trade Academy Natural Hair Care staff: Ms. Marion, Ms. Jones, CJ, and Aunt Bert. Thanks for the encouragement and support that helped me pass the written and practical state board exams on the first try.

To my amazing classmates, Kenielle, Ayanna, Ebony, and Monica, I learned from each of you.

To Shennan Scott, thank you for inviting me to work at your salon. It inspired me to see myself as more than a hobbyist. It put me on the path to "get legal" ;-) It changed the course of my life.

To my locking mentor, Kris McDred, thank you for putting out that first youtube video. I was one of the millions that watched it many years ago and used it to instant loc, my first client. Who knew I'd get to learn directly from the source? Thank you for encouraging us all to master locking.

To Rob Fitzpatrick, Adam Rosen, and the Monday and Wednesday Writing Accountability Group members. You pushed me to outdo what I did last, lol. I may have quit if I didn't know you all might miss my reports ;-)

To Mike Capuzzi, your books and podcast were my guides along the way. I am looking forward to working with you on a future book.

To Matt Rudnitsky, your book allowed me to stop making excuses and finish the thing!

To my beta readers: Zoe French, Victoria Lee, Shavonna Haamid, Kenielle Jefferies, and Monica Lavice I really appreciate you taking the time to look over the book and give feedback to make it better.

If I missed anyone, count it to my head and not my heart, and let me know so I can update the next edition!

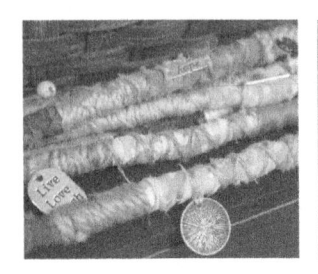

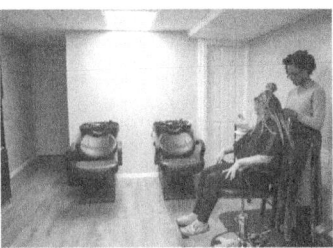

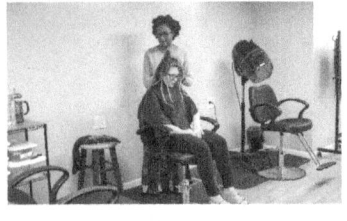

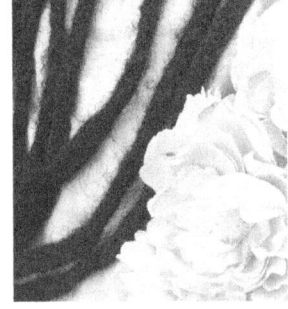

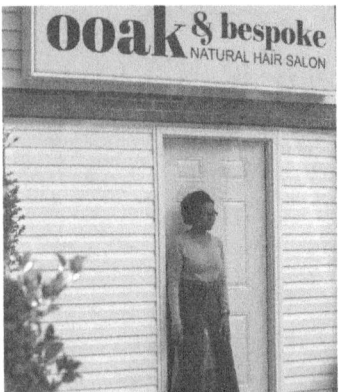

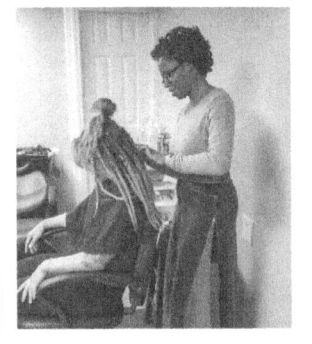

Model: Kristy Marshal
Photographer: Erin Hardy, Hardy Photography

About Amy McKnight

Amy McKnight is a Licensed Natural Hair Care Specialist and Loctician living in Lexington, North Carolina. She specializes in hard-to-lock hair types, instant loc, and loc extension installations, and interlock loc installation and maintenance. She creates customized lock installation and maintenance plans based on her client's lifestyles, hair types, and ultimate goals for having locs.

She has had natural locks or worn some type of faux loc style on and off for over 20 years. She was an editor and the main contributor for MyNHCG.com, formally N aturalHairCareGuide.com, where she wrote dozens of articles on locs and hair locking.

Amy has done hair on and off as a side business for over a decade. When she learned that licensing is required to do hair in North Carolina, where she resides, she returned to school to get the required certification. She then opened a state-licensed 2-chair salon, OOAK & Bespoke Natural Hair Salon.

Before making the career switch to entirely focus on loc care, she taught creative rigid heddle weaving on and offline. She enjoys fiber arts and yarn crafting and loves being able to bring that background into what she does with her clients.

She and her husband Conrad own a successful computer repair and sales business. She worked there for ten years before switching careers to open her salon. They have one daughter, one dog, one guinea pig, four gerbils, and three freshwater fish.

Also By Amy McKnight

Dreadful Beauty

Interlock Love (Coming 2023)

*Tendrilocs: Next Generation Micro-Sized Braid Locs
(Coming 2023)*

About the Freedom In Locs Podcast

The *Freedom in Locs Podcast* is an interview-style podcast with host Amy McKnight, locticians, women who wear locs, and businesses who support them.

Each episode shares information, encouragement, and support for women who wear, want, or love locs. If you are looking for a virtual community to encourage you tune into the show!

Listen on Spotify. Just type in "Freedom In Locs"

A Small Request

Thank you so much for reading *Freedom In Locs*! I'm positive that if you follow this book's information, you will be on your way to having amazingly beautiful locs. If you have any questions or want to tell me what you think about *Freedom in Locs,* email me at OOAKandBespoke@gmail.com. I'd love to hear from you!

When you do, please send me a selfie. I'd love to see how your locs came out!

I have a small, quick favor to ask. Would you mind taking a minute or two and sending me an honest review of this book? Reviews are the BEST way to help others find out about this book, and I read all my reviews looking for helpful feedback. Visit:

OOAKandBespoke.com/books

Click the book's name, and you'll see a link to leave a review! Thank you in advance!

Made in the USA
Columbia, SC
08 October 2022